94 Acne Clearing Meal and Juice Recipes:

The Fast and Natural Path to Resolving Your Acne Problems

By

Joe Correa CSN

COPYRIGHT

This publication is designed to provide accurate and authoritative information in regard to the subject matter covered. It is sold with the understanding that neither the author nor the publisher is engaged in rendering medical advice. If medical advice or assistance is needed, consult with a doctor. This book is considered a guide and should not be used in any way detrimental to your health. Consult with a physician before starting this nutritional plan to make sure it's right for you.

ACKNOWLEDGEMENTS

This book is dedicated to my friends and family that have had mild or serious illnesses so that you may find a solution and make the necessary changes in your life.

94 Acne Clearing Meal and Juice Recipes:

The Fast and Natural Path to Resolving Your Acne Problems

By

Joe Correa CSN

CONTENTS

ABOUT THE AUTHOR

After years of Research, I honestly believe in the positive effects that proper nutrition can have over the body and mind. My knowledge and experience has helped me live healthier throughout the years and which I have shared with family and friends. The more you know about eating and drinking healthier, the sooner you will want to change your life and eating habits.

Nutrition is a key part in the process of being healthy and living longer so get started today. The first step is the most important and the most significant.

INTRODUCTION

94 Acne Clearing Meal and Juice Recipes: The Fast and Natural Path to Resolving Your Acne Problems

By Joe Correa CSN

In order to cure both: the hormonal imbalance that causes acne, and to heal your skin once and for all, you will have to dig a little further into what the real problem is. Studies have shown that the lack of nutrients such as omega 3 fatty acids, carbohydrates, vitamins, and other antioxidants is the real cause.

Healthy and nutritional diets are a universal cure and the true prevention of acne. For example, some foods increase blood sugar, that in turn releases a hormone called insulin. This hormone is responsible for the increase of oil production in our skin which causes those terrible bumps on the skin. But, by maintaining a healthy diet, you can keep your blood sugar in balance and prevent high oil production on your skin.

I have created this book with acne-specific recipes based on healthy ingredients that are proven antioxidants, high in omega 3 fatty acids, and full of healthy fruits and vegetables in lots of different combinations.

Acne is often treated with drugs and cosmetic products making it a very profitable industry worldwide. However, these products often don't cure acne the way they should. They temporarily cure the visible part but don't create a significant affect on the cause of this condition.

Let these meal and juice recipes be your guide to getting rid of acne once and for all. Eat and drink the right foods to bring back healthy and beautiful skin!

94 ACNE CLEARING MEAL AND JUICE RECIPES: THE FAST AND NATURAL PATH TO RESOLVING YOUR ACNE PROBLEMS

MEALS

1.　Orange Rice Salad

Ingredients:

1 cup of white rice, pre-cooked

1 large orange, peeled and wedged

1 large bell pepper, chopped

2 tbsp of lemon juice

2 tbsp of sour cream

1 tbsp of olive oil

1 tsp of fresh parsley, finely chopped

¼ tsp of salt

4 lettuce leaves

Preparation:

Combine sour cream, lemon juice, oil, parsley, and salt in a mixing bowl. Stir well and set aside.

Place rice in a deep pot. Add 3 cups of water and bring it to a boil. Cook until water evaporates, or until set. Set aside to cool completely.

Now, combine rice and pepper in a large salad bowl. Drizzle with dressing and stir all well.

Place lettuce leaves on serving plates and spoon the mixture into equal portions.

Nutrition information per serving: Kcal: 245, Protein: 4.3g, Carbs: 45.2g, Fats: 5.3g

2.   Lemon Salmon

Ingredients:

2 lbs of salmon filets, skinless and boneless

2 medium-sized lemons, sliced

½ cup of lemon juice, freshly squeezed

1 tbsp of olive oil

1 tbsp of rosemary, finely chopped

¼ tsp of black pepper, freshly ground

1 tbsp of sour cream

Preparation:

Combine lemon juice, sour cream, olive oil, rosemary, salt, and pepper in small a mixing bowl. Stir all well and set aside to allow flavors to mingle.

Take a large nonstick baking dish and make a fine layer of lemon slices. Top with filets and drizzle all with marinade.

Put it in the oven and bake for about 13-15 minutes, or until set. Serve with fresh vegetables.

Nutrition information per serving: Kcal: 347, Protein: 44.4g, Carbs: 1.4g, Fats: 18.5g

3. Green Soup

Ingredients:

2 lbs of asparagus, trimmed

1 cup of fresh spinach, finely chopped

5 cups of skim milk

1 cup of chicken broth

2 tbsp of butter

2 tbsp of all-purpose flour

½ tsp of salt

¼ tsp of black pepper, ground

Preparation:

Combine milk and chicken broth in a large saucepan over a medium-high temperature. Add asparagus and spinach and bring it to a boil. Cook for about 10-15 minutes, or until soften. Remove from the heat and transfer asparagus and spinach to a food processor. Reserve the saucepan with milk and broth mixture.

Blend until smooth and set aside.

Melt the butter in a frying pan over a medium-high temperature. Add flour and cook until golden. Pour in the saucepan with milk mixture and stir well. Add blended asparagus and spinach. Stir once again and bring it to a boil. Sprinkle with some salt and pepper to taste.

Serve warm.

Nutrition information per serving: Kcal: 94, Protein: 6.8g, Carbs: 10.9g, Fats: 2.6g

4.   Kefir Meat Balls

Ingredients:

1 lb of minced beef

1 large onion, peeled and finely chopped

1 tbsp of fresh rosemary, finely chopped

1 large egg

¼ cup of kefir cream

2 tbsp of all-purpose flour

½ tsp of salt

¼ tsp of black pepper, ground

1 tbsp of vegetable oil

For the topping:

2 cups of kefir

3 garlic cloves, crushed

1 tbsp of fresh rosemary, finely chopped

¼ tsp of salt

Preparation:

Combine the ingredients in a large bowl. Add about two tablespoons of oil in the mixture and shape the meatballs using your hands.

Heat up some oil in a large skillet, over a medium-high temperature. Fry the meatballs for about 10 minutes, or until lightly charred. Remove from the heat and allow it to cool.

Combine two cups of kefir with crushed garlic and fresh rosemary. Top the meatballs with it.

These meatballs are best cold. I suggest you keep them in the refrigerator overnight.

Nutrition information per serving: Kcal: 502, Protein: 31.2g, Carbs: 8.0g, Fats: 38.4g

5. Chia Blueberry Smoothie

Ingredients:

1 cup of almond milk, unsweetened

½ medium-sized banana, sliced

1 cup of frozen blueberries

¼ cup of dates, pitted and chopped

1 tbsp of chia seeds

A few mint leaves

Preparation:

Combine milk, banana, blueberries, and dates in a food processor. Blend until smooth. Add water to adjust a thickness of the mixture and re-blend if needed.

Transfer the mixture to the serving glasses and top with chia seeds and fresh mint leaves.

Nutrition information per serving: Kcal: 281, Protein: 3.1g, Carbs: 29.5g, Fats: 19.7g

6.   Eggplant Casserole

Ingredients:

2 large eggplants, diced

2 small onions, diced

1 medium-sized bell pepper, cubed

7 garlic cloves, minced

2 medium-sized tomatoes, diced

1 cup of fresh basil, chopped

½ tsp of salt

¼ tsp of black pepper, freshly ground

Preparation:

Preheat the oven to 375°F.

Place the onions in a large nonstick saucepan over a medium-high temperature. Stir-fry for about 8-10 minutes, or until translucent. Add garlic, pepper, eggplant and about 1-2 tablespoons of water. Reduce the heat to low, cover with a lid and cook for 15 minutes. Add tomatoes and sprinkle with some salt and pepper to taste. Cook for another 10 minutes, then add basil. Stir well and remove from the heat.

Transfer the mixture to a casserole dish. Put it in the oven and bake for about 25-30 minutes, or until heated trough.

Nutrition information per serving: Kcal: 75, Protein: 3.0g, Carbs: 17.3g, Fats: 0.5g

7. Avocado Spinach Salad

Ingredients:

1 medium-sized avocado, peeled, pitted, and cubed

1 cup of fresh spinach, chopped

1 cup of Iceberg lettuce, chopped

1 medium-sized carrot, grated

1 large egg, hard-boiled, wedged

1 tbsp of lemon juice

1 tbsp of olive oil

½ tsp of salt

½ tsp of black pepper, ground

Preparation:

Mix together lemon juice, oil, salt, and pepper in a mixing bowl. Toss well and set aside.

Combine avocado, spinach, lettuce, carrot, and egg in a large salad bowl. Drizzle with dressing and stir well. Serve immediately.

Nutrition information per serving: Kcal: 324, Protein: 6.0g, Carbs: 13.7g, Fats: 29.3g

8.   Banana Dates Parfait

Ingredients:

2 medium-sized bananas, sliced

½ cup of dates, pitted and chopped

8 oz of Greek yogurt

2 tbsp of skim milk

2 tbsp of lemon juice

1 tsp of vanilla extract

1 cup of rolled oats, cooked

Preparation:

Place the rolled oats in a small pot of boiling water. Cook for 3-4 minutes and remove from the heat. Drain and set aside.

Combine yogurt, milk, lemon juice, vanilla extract, and one banana in a food processor. Blend until nicely smooth.

In a serving glass, spoon one layer of the banana mixture, then add few dates and banana slices. Repeat the process with remaining ingredients until done.

Refrigerate 1 hour before serving. Garnish with some extra fruit before serving.

Nutrition information per serving: Kcal: 243, Protein: 9.9g, Carbs: 47.0g, Fats: 2.8g

9.   Tuna with Mashed Cauliflower

Ingredients:

5 oz of tuna filets, skinless and boneless

1 large cauliflower head, chopped

2 garlic cloves, minced

1 tbsp of olive oil

¼ cup of cream cheese

1 tbsp of lemon juice, freshly squeezed

½ tsp of sea salt

¼ tsp of black pepper, ground

Preparation:

Place the cauliflower in a pot of boiling water. Cook for about 10-15 minutes, or until fork-tender. Remove from the heat and drain well. Set aside.

Transfer the cauliflower to a food processor. Add cheese and garlic and blend until smooth.

Preheat the oil in a large skillet over a medium-high temperature. Add filets and cook for 5 minutes on each side, or until set. remove from the heat and serve with mashed cauliflower. Drizzle with lemon juice. Enjoy!

Nutrition information per serving: Kcal: 333, Protein: 23.9g, Carbs: 9.1g, Fats: 23.1g

10.   Black Beans with Brown Rice

Ingredients:

4 cups of black beans, pre-cooked

3 cups of brown rice, pre-cooked

5 garlic cloves, minced

2 small onions, chopped

1 red bell pepper, diced

1 tsp of cumin, ground

1 small chili pepper, chopped

1 tsp of oregano, ground

½ tsp of salt

¼ tsp of black pepper, ground

Preparation:

Place the rice in a deep pot. add 5 cups of water and cook until water evaporates, or until set. Set aside to cool.

Combine pepper, onions, chili, and 2 tablespoons of water in a large saucepan over a medium-high temperature. Cook for 10 minutes and then add garlic, oregano, and cumin. Stir well and cook for another 2-3 minutes.

Add the beans and 1 cup of water. Sprinkle with salt and pepper and cook for 10 minutes more. Remove from the heat and let it cool for a while.

Serve with beans and rice with lemon slices and sprinkle with some extra salt and pepper if needed. Enjoy!

Nutrition information per serving: Kcal: 484, Protein: 21.5g, Carbs: 94.7g, Fats: 2.7g

11. Turkey with Avocado and Cucumber

Ingredients:

2 lbs of turkey breasts, skinless and boneless, chopped

1 small avocado, peeled, pitted, diced

1 large cucumber, sliced

2 tbsp of olive oil

1 tbsp of lemon juice

½ tsp of salt

¼ tsp of black pepper, freshly ground

Preparation:

Preheat the oil in a large nonstick saucepan over a medium-high temperature. Add turkey and cook for about 10-15 minutes or until nicely browned. Remove from the heat and set aside.

Combine avocado and cucumber in a medium bowl. Sprinkle with salt, pepper, and rosemary to taste. Toss well and transfer to a serving plate, together with meat. Drizzle with lemon juice.

Nutrition information per serving: Kcal: 274, Protein: 26.8g, Carbs: 11.2g, Fats: 13.8g

12.   Basil Veggie Pasta

Ingredients:

12 oz of pasta, whole-grain

1 lb of artichokes, halved

1 cup of cherry tomato, halved

1 cup of fresh basil, chopped

½ tsp of salt

¼ tsp of black pepper, ground

2 tbsp of sour cream

1 tbsp of fresh parsley, finely chopped

Preparation:

Cook pasta using package instructions. Drain well and set aside.

Combine artichokes, tomatoes, and basil in a large bowl. Sprinkle with salt and pepper and toss well. Add pasta and stir all together.

Combine sour cream and parsley and stir well. Pour over the pasta and vegetable mixture and give it a good stir. Serve immediately.

Nutrition information per serving: Kcal: 211, Protein: 9.2g, Carbs: 39.7g, Fats: 2.3g

13.　Avocado Eggs with Cranberries

Ingredients:

2 large eggs, hard-boiled

1 small avocado, pitted, peeled, and chopped

1 cup of cucumber, cut into bite-sized pieces

¼ cup of fresh cranberries

1 medium-sized tomato, diced

1 tbsp of parsley, finely chopped

Preparation:

Combine avocado, cucumber, and tomato in a food processor. Blend until smooth mixture and set aside.

Cut the eggs in wedges and place them on a serving plate. Pour over the previously made mixture. Top with cranberries and serve.

Nutrition information per serving: Kcal: 202, Protein: 6.1g, Carbs: 9.8g, Fats: 16.5g

14.   Sweet Potato Beef Stew

Ingredients:

1 large sweet potato, peeled and chopped

1 lb of lean beef, skinless, boneless, chopped

3 cups of vegetable broth

1 small onion, diced

1 large carrot, sliced

2 small zucchinis, peeled and sliced

1 red bell pepper, chopped

1 tsp of dried thyme, ground

2 garlic cloves, minced

1 tbsp of olive oil

½ tsp of salt

¼ tsp of black pepper, ground

Preparation:

Place the potatoes in a pot of boiling water. Cook for 10 minutes, or until slightly soften. Remove from the heat and drain. Set aside.

Preheat the oil in a slow cooker over a medium-high temperature. Add onion and garlic and stir-fry until translucent. Add carrot, zucchinis, bell pepper, and 1 cup of water. Cook until water evaporates.

Now, add all other ingredients and reduce the heat to low. Cover with a lid and cook for 4-5 hours. Adjust the thickness of the stew adding more water.

Serve warm.

Nutrition information per serving: Kcal: 231, Protein: 27.0g, Carbs: 12.3g, Fats: 7.9g

15.   Bulgur Tomatoes

Ingredients:

4 large tomatoes, whole

1 cup of fresh leeks, diced

1 small zucchini, diced

1 medium-sized carrot, diced

1 cup of bulgur, pre-cooked

2 cups of vegetable broth

1 cup of fresh basil, finely chopped

¼ cup of lemon juice

¼ tsp of salt

¼ tsp of black pepper, ground

Preparation:

Preheat the oven to 375°F.

Combine bulgur and vegetable broth in a large pot. Bring it to a boil and cook for 10 minutes. Stir occasionally. Remove from the heat and drain. Set aside to cool.

Scoop the tomatoes and reserve the flesh. Set aside.

Combine leeks and garlic in a large nonstick saucepan over a medium-high temperature. Cook for about 5-6 minutes, stirring constantly. Add bulgur, lemon juice, and basil. Sprinkle with salt and pepper and stir all well. Cook for another 3-4 minutes and remove from the heat.

Spoon this mixture into tomatoes, and place them in a large baking dish. Cover and bake for 30 minutes. Serve warm.

Nutrition information per serving: Kcal: 284, Protein: 6.3g, Carbs: 26.9g, Fats: 1.2g

16.   Beans and Onions Wraps

Ingredients:

2 cups of kidney beans, pre-cooked, drained and rinsed

1 large bell pepper, finely chopped

¼ cup of fresh parsley, finely chopped

1 small red onion, finely chopped

3 oz of Greek yogurt

1 tbsp of olive oil

1 tbsp of lemon juice

3 lettuce leaves

Preparation:

Place the beans in a large pot over a medium-high temperature. Add 4 cups of water and cook until soften. Remove from the heat. Drain and rinse well.

Mix together yogurt, lemon juice, and olive oil in a mixing bowl. Set aside.

Now, combine cooked beans, pepper, parsley, and onion in a large bowl. Drizzle with dressing and toss well.

Spoon the mixture into lettuce leaves and secure with a lid. Refrigerate for 30 minutes before serving.

Nutrition information per serving: Kcal: 500, Protein: 31.2g, Carbs: 81.9g, Fats: 6.7g

17.   Cucumber Tomato Salad

Ingredients:

1 medium-sized cucumber, sliced

1 cup of cherry tomatoes, halved

1 cup of Feta cheese, crumbled

2 tbsp of extra virgin olive oil

1 tbsp of balsamic vinegar

2 tbsp of lemon juice

1 tsp of vegetable seasoning mix

¼ tsp of salt

1 tsp of fresh rosemary, finely chopped

¼ tsp of black pepper, ground

1 tbsp of fresh parsley, finely chopped

Preparation:

Mix together oil, vinegar, lemon juice, vegetable seasoning mix, rosemary, salt, and pepper in a small bowl. Stir well and set aside to allow flavors to meld.

Combine cucumber, cherry tomatoes, and cheese in a large bowl. Drizzle with dressing and toss well to combine. Sprinkle with fresh parsley and serve immediately.

Nutrition information per serving: Kcal: 183, Protein: 6.3g, Carbs: 6.5g, Fats: 15.3g

18.   Grilled Tuna with Peppers

Ingredients:

1 lb of tuna filets, skinless and boneless

4 large bell peppers, cut into strips

1 small onion, sliced

3 tbsp of olive oil

1 tbsp of lemon juice

1 tbsp of orange juice

½ tsp of salt

¼ tsp of black pepper, ground

1 tsp of fresh rosemary, finely chopped

2 garlic cloves, minced

Preparation:

Combine lemon juice, orange juice, rosemary, and 2 tablespoons of olive oil in a large marinade bowl. Add filets and refrigerate for 30 minutes to allow flavors to penetrate into the meat.

Preheat the remaining oil in a large nonstick skillet over a medium-high temperature. Add onion and garlic and stir-fry until translucent. Add bell peppers and cook for 10 minutes or until crisp-tender. Remove the peppers and reserve the pan. Add tuna filets and cook for about 4-5 minutes on each side. Remove from the heat and serve with peppers. Drizzle with remaining marinade.

Nutrition information per serving: Kcal: 352, Protein: 31.7g, Carbs: 11.9g, Fats: 20.1g

19.   White Bean Soup

Ingredients:

2 cups of white beans, pre-cooked

6 garlic cloves, minced

1 medium-sized onion, diced

2 medium-sized potatoes, peeled and chopped

1 cup of fresh kale, chopped

4 cups of vegetable broth

½ tsp of salt

¼ tsp of black pepper, ground

1 tbsp of sour cream

1 tsp of vegetable oil

Preparation:

Preheat the oil in a deep pot over a medium-high temperature. Add the onion and stir-fry for 5 minutes, or until translucent. Add garlic and about 2 tablespoons of water and continue to cook for another 2 minutes.

Add vegetable broth, kale, beans, and potatoes. Reduce the temperature to low and cover with a lid. Cook for about 45-50 minutes, or until beans soften.

Stir in the sour cream and sprinkle with salt and pepper to taste. Cook for another 5 minutes, stirring constantly.

Nutrition information per serving: Kcal: 246, Protein: 15.7g, Carbs: 42.3g, Fats: 2.1g

20.   Green Tropical Smoothie

Ingredients:

2 cups of fresh spinach, roughly chopped

1 cup of pineapple, chopped

1 cup of mango, chopped

1 cup of coconut milk

1 tbsp of Brazil nuts

Preparation:

Place spinach in a pot of boiling water. Cook for 2 minutes and remove from the heat. Set aside to cool.

Now, combine spinach and fruits in a food processor and blend. Add coconut water and few ice cubes and re-blend.

Transfer the mixture to a serving glasses and top with Brazil nuts.

Nutrition information per serving: Kcal: 348, Protein: 5.1g, Carbs: 30.3g, Fats: 26.3g

21.　Salmon Mushroom Wraps

Ingredients:

1 lb of salmon, cut into bite-sized pieces

1 lb of button mushrooms, chopped

2 medium-sized bell peppers, chopped

1 cup of frozen corn, thawed

1 small red onion, chopped

2 tbsp of olive oil

1 tbsp of lemon juice

1 tsp of dried rosemary, finely chopped

1 tsp of sea salt

½ tsp of black pepper, ground

6 lettuce leaves

Preparation:

Preheat the oil in a large skillet over a medium-high temperature. Add mushrooms, peppers, and onion. Cook for 10 minutes or until soften, stirring constantly. Add meat and sprinkle with salt and pepper to taste. Cook for 10 minutes more. Add corn, lemon juice, and rosemary. Stir well to combine and cook for another 2-3 minutes. Remove from the heat and let it cool.

Spread lettuce leaves on serving plates. Spoon the mixture and wrap. Secure with a toothpick. You can add 1 tablespoon of tomato sauce or sour cream. This is, however, optional.

Nutrition information per serving: Kcal: 197, Protein: 18.4g, Carbs: 11.7g, Fats: 10.0g

22. Pumpkin Almond Smoothie

Ingredients:

1 cup of pumpkin, peeled and cubed

1 cup of almond milk

¼ cup of dates, pitted and chopped

½ tsp of vanilla extract

¼ tsp of cinnamon, ground

1 tbsp of flaxseeds

Preparation:

Combine all ingredients in a food processor. Blend until smooth and transfer to a serving glasses. Refrigerate for 1 hour before serving.

Nutrition information per serving: Kcal: 227, Protein: 3.2g, Carbs: 11.9g, Fats: 20.0g

23.   Grilled Juicy Beef

Ingredients:

4 lbs of beef steaks, boneless

1 cup of tomato sauce

2 small onions, diced

1 cup of fresh celery, diced

1 cup of button mushrooms, chopped

1 cup of water

2 tbsp of all-purpose flour

3 tbsp of olive oil

½ tsp of chili pepper, ground

Preparation:

Preheat the oil in a large skillet over a medium-high temperature. Add the onions and stir-fry until translucent. Add meat and pour the tomato sauce. Reduce the heat to low and cover with a lid. Simmer for 1 hour until soften.

Add mushrooms and celery. Cook for another 20 minutes.

Meanwhile, combine flour, sour cream, water, salt, and pepper in a nonstick pan over a medium-temperature. Stir and cook for 2 minutes constantly until the mixture thickens.

Stir in this mixture into the pan with meat and cook for 5 minutes more. Remove from the heat and serve.

Nutrition information per serving: Kcal: 393, Protein: 56.0g, Carbs: 4.4g, Fats: 15.6g

24.　Baked Potatoes with Onions & Peppers

Ingredients:

5 large potatoes, peeled and halved

1 medium-sized onion, sliced

1 cup of red bell peppers, chopped

1 cup of spring onions, chopped

1 garlic clove, minced

½ tsp of cumin, ground

¼ tsp of salt

¼ tsp of Cayenne pepper, ground

2 tbsp of olive oil

Preparation:

Preheat the oven to 375°F.

Grease a large baking sheet with 1 tablespoon of oil. Spread the potatoes and pierce them with a fork. Sprinkle with salt and cayenne pepper and put it in the oven. Bake for 1 hour, or until nicely soften. Remove from the heat and let it cool for a while.

Meanwhile, preheat the remaining oil in a large saucepan over a medium-high temperature. Add onion, spring onions, and garlic. Cook for 5 minutes, or until onions translucent. Now, add 2 tablespoons of water, cumin, and a pinch of salt. Cook for about 3-4 minutes more, stirring constantly. Remove from the heat.

Pour the onion mixture over the potatoes and serve. You can top with a tablespoon of sour cream. However, this is optional.

Nutrition information per serving: Kcal: 164, Protein: 3.6g, Carbs: 31.8g, Fats: 3.1g

25.   Strawberry Flaxseeds Smoothie

Ingredients:

1 cup of strawberries, chopped

1 large peach, pitted and chopped

1 cup of skim milk

1 tbsp of flaxseeds

Preparation:

Combine all ingredients in a food processor. Blend until nicely smooth and transfer to a serving glasses. Refrigerate for 1 hour before serving.

Nutrition information per serving: Kcal: 116, Protein: 5.8g, Carbs: 19.5g, Fats: 1.5g

26.   Spinach Quinoa Pilaf

Ingredients:

4 cups of baby spinach, chopped

1 lb of button mushrooms, pre-cooked and chopped

2 cups of leeks, diced

2 garlic cloves, minced

2 cups of vegetable broth

1 cup of white quinoa, pre-cooked

½ tsp of salt

¼ tsp of dried thyme, ground

¼ tsp of black pepper, ground

1 tbsp of vegetable oil

Preparation:

Place mushrooms in a large pot and pour enough water to cover. Cook until soften and remove from the heat. Set aside.

Add 2 cups of water to a deep pot and bring it to a boil. Add quinoa and cook for 5 minutes. Remove from the heat and drain. Set aside.

Preheat the oil in a large nonstick saucepan over a medium-high temperature. Add leeks and mushrooms. Cook for about 8-10 minutes, stirring constantly. Stir in garlic and thyme and cook for another minute. Add vegetable broth, quinoa, and spinach. Reduce the heat and cover with a lid.

Cook for about 15-20 minutes. Sprinkle with salt and pepper and give it a good stir. Remove from the heat and serve.

Nutrition information per serving: Kcal: 135, Protein: 7.8g, Carbs: 22.6g, Fats: 2.2g

27.   Apple Acorn Squash Soup

Ingredients:

1 large acorn squash, peeled, seeded, and cut into bite-sized pieces

2 large apples, peeled and chopped

1tbsp of curry powder

1 small onion, diced

2 tbsp of apple cider vinegar

3 cups of vegetable broth

¼ tsp of Cayenne pepper

¼ tsp of black pepper, ground

½ tsp of salt

Preparation:

Place the onion in a large nonstick skillet over a medium-high temperature. Stir-fry for 10 minutes, or until translucent. Now, add vegetable broth, acorn squash, vinegar, curry, and 2 tablespoons of water to the pan. Reduce the heat to low and cover with a lid. Cook until acorn squash soften. Remove from the heat and let it cool for a few minutes.

Transfer the mixture to a food processor. Blend until smooth and return to the pot to reheat. Sprinkle with salt and cayenne pepper to taste.

Serve warm.

Nutrition information per serving: Kcal: 96, Protein: 3.5g, Carbs: 20.1g, Fats: 1.1g

28.   Mussels with Veggies

Ingredients:

10 oz of shelled mussels

1 small carrot, diced

1 small onion, chopped

1 medium-sized bell pepper, chopped

2 small potatoes, peeled and chopped

1 cup of fresh parsley, finely chopped

2 small tomatoes, diced

2 tbsp of flaxseed oil

½ tsp of salt

¼ tsp of black pepper, ground

Preparation:

Place potatoes in a pot of boiling water and cook for 3 minutes. remove from the heat and set aside.

Preheat the oil in a large nonstick saucepan over a medium-high temperature. Add tomatoes, carrot, pepper, onion, and parsley. Stir well and cook for 10 minutes, or until veggies slightly soften. Stir in mussels and sprinkle with some salt and pepper to taste. Cover with a lid and cook for about 5-7 minutes more, or until set.

Remove from the heat and serve with pasta or rice. This is, however, optional.

Nutrition information per serving: Kcal: 159, Protein: 2.9g, Carbs: 21.3g, Fats: 7.4g

29.   Cranberry Orange Cookies

Ingredients:

1 cup of orange juice

2 cups of all-purpose flour

½ cup of almond butter

¼ cup of apple sauce

2 tsp of baking powder

1 tbsp of cornstarch

1 tsp of salt

2 tbsp of flaxseeds

¼ cup of dried cranberries

1 tsp of vanilla extract

Preparation:

Preheat the oven to 375°F.

Combine all dry ingredients in a large bowl. Add applesauce, vanilla extract and orange juice. Blend all using a hand mixer. Set aside.

Place some baking paper on a large baking sheet. Form the balls or bars and spread over a baking sheet. Place it in the oven and bake for 25 minutes, or until golden brown. Remove from the oven and let it cool for a while.

Serve some melted dark chocolate with the cookies. However, this is optional.

Nutrition information per serving: Kcal: 82, Protein: 2.1g, Carbs: 16.0g, Fats: 0.8g

30.   Raspberry Omelet

Ingredients:

3 egg whites

3 free-range eggs

½ cup of raspberries

2 tbsp of tartar sauce

2 tbsp of butter

½ tsp of salt

¼ tsp of black pepper, ground

Preparation:

Combine egg whites and tartar sauce in a mixing bowl. Sprinkle with salt and pepper to taste and whisk with a fork. Set aside.

In a separate bowl, combine eggs and raspberries. Mix to combine and set aside.

Melt the butter in a large nonstick frying pan over a medium-high temperature. pour the raspberry egg mixture and cook for 2 minutes. Add egg white mixture and continue to cook for another 3-4 minutes. Flip the omelet and cook for 2 minutes. Remove from the heat and fold with a spatula.

Serve immediately.

Nutrition information per serving: Kcal: 309, Protein: 14.2g, Carbs: 7.7g, Fats: 25.4g

31.   Salmon Pepper Boats

Ingredients:

4 medium-sized bell peppers, seeded and halved

1 lb of salmon, cut into bite-sized pieces

2 medium-sized potatoes, mashed

½ cup of corn, kernels removed

½ tsp of dry rosemary, ground

½ tsp of salt

¼ tsp of black pepper, ground

1 tbsp of oil

Preparation:

Preheat the oil in a large nonstick pan over a medium-high temperature. Add salmon chops and cook for about 10 minutes or until golden, stirring constantly.

Place the potatoes in a pot of boiling water. Cook until fork-tender and remove from the heat. Drain well and set aside to cool completely. Place the potatoes in a food processor and add blend until smooth. Transfer the mixture to large bowl and stir in the corn, and some salt and pepper to taste.

Spoon the potato mixture into the pepper halves and top with salmon. Sprinkle with rosemary and serve.

Nutrition information per serving: Kcal: 154, Protein: 12.8g, Carbs: 14.8g, Fats: 5.5g

32. Peanut Butter Banana Smoothie

Ingredients:

1 tbsp of peanut butter

2 medium-sized bananas, chopped

1 cup of skim milk

¼ cup of dates, pitted and chopped

1 tsp of cocoa powder

1 tbsp of dark chocolate, melted

Preparation:

Combine all ingredients in a food processor and blend until nicely smooth. Transfer the mixture to a serving glasses. Top with melted chocolate and refrigerate for 20 minutes before serving.

Nutrition information per serving: Kcal: 193, Protein: 5.6g, Carbs: 36.6g, Fats: 4.1g

33. Orange Black Bean Salad

Ingredients:

5 large oranges, peeled and roughly chopped

4 cups of arugula, finely chopped

1 cup of fennel, trimmed and chopped

2 cups of black beans, pre-cooked

¼ tsp of salt

2 tbsp of olive oil

1 tbsp of balsamic vinegar

¼ tsp of black pepper, ground

¼ tsp of Cayenne pepper, ground

Preparation:

Place the beans in a pot of boiling water. Cook until soften and remove from the heat. Drain well and set aside.

Mix together oil, vinegar, cayenne pepper, salt, and pepper in a small mixing bowl. Toss well and set aside.

Now, combine arugula, fennel, and beans in a large salad bowl. Drizzle with previously made dressing and toss well to coat. Let it stand for 15 minutes before serving to allow flavors to mingle.

Enjoy!

Nutrition information per serving: Kcal: 256, Protein: 12.0g, Carbs: 45.0g, Fats: 4.4g

34.   Sea Bass Stew

Ingredients:

4 sea bass filets, skinless and boneless

4 small onions, chopped

2 garlic cloves, minced

1 cup of parsley, finely chopped

4 cherry tomatoes, diced

¼ cup of green olives, pitted and chopped

2 tbsp of olive oil

1 tbsp of balsamic vinegar

1 tsp of lemon zest, freshly grated

1 tsp of chili pepper, ground

Preparation:

Preheat the oil in a large nonstick saucepan over a medium-high temperature. Add onions and stir-fry until translucent. Stir in diced cherry tomatoes and olives. Cook for about 10-15 minutes. Remove from the heat.

Pour half of the tomato mixture in a deep pot. Make a layer of meat and top with remaining tomato mixture. Stir in the vinegar and sprinkle with lemon zest, chilli pepper, and parsley. Reduce the heat and cover with a lid.

Cook for about 20 minutes and remove the lid. Stir the stew couple of times and add extra salt if needed. Cook for 5 minutes and remove from the heat.

Serve warm.

Nutrition information per serving: Kcal: 173, Protein: 17.6g, Carbs: 9.4g, Fats: 7.6g

35.   Greek Yogurt Soup

Ingredients:

1 cup of white rice, pre-cooked

1 lb of Greek yogurt

2 oz of butter

1 tsp of chili pepper, ground

½ tsp of salt

Preparation:

Place the rice in a deep pot. Add 2 cups of water and cook for 20 minutes, or until set. Remove from the heat and let it cool.

Combine rice and yogurt in a food processor. Blend until smooth. Transfer to a serving bowl.

Melt the butter in a saucepan and add chili pepper. Drizzle the soup with this mixture. Sprinkle with salt and serve.

Nutrition information per serving: Kcal: 357, Protein: 14.9g, Carbs: 41.7g, Fats: 14.1g

36.   Creamy Beef Balls

Ingredients:

1 lb of minced beef

½ cup of fresh parsley, finely chopped

1 small onion, finely chopped

1 tsp of cumin, ground

1 tbsp of olive oil

2 slices of bread

2 tbsp of cream cheese

Preparation:

Soak the bread slices in water for 5 minutes. drain and squeeze the water and transfer it to a large bowl. Add meat, onion, cumin, parsley, salt, and pepper. Mix all squeezing with hands.

Form the ball-shaped pieces with oil-greased hands.

Preheat the oil in a large nonstick frying pan and fry the balls for about 5-7 minutes or until nicely brown. Transfer the balls to a serving plate. Top with cream cheese.

Nutrition information per serving: Kcal: 270, Protein: 35.7g, Carbs: 5.1g, Fats: 11.0g

37.   Green Salad with Greek Yogurt Dressing

Ingredients:

3 cups of Romaine lettuce, chopped

1 large apple, cored and chopped

½ cup of spring onions, chopped

1 large bell pepper, chopped

2 tbsp of almonds, roughly chopped

For the dressing:

¼ cup of Greek yogurt

3 tbsp of olive oil

2 tbsp of balsamic vinegar

¼ tsp of salt

¼ tsp of black pepper, ground

Preparation:

Combine all dressing ingredients in a mixing bowl and toss well. Set aside to allow flavor to meld.

In a large salad bowl, mix lettuce, apple, onions, and pepper. Drizzle the salad with dressing and top with almonds. Add extra salt and pepper to taste, if needed.

Nutrition information per serving: Kcal: 157, Protein: 1.5g, Carbs: 12.9g, Fats: 12.3g

38.   Orange Carrot Smoothe

Ingredients:

2 large oranges, chopped

1 large carrot, chopped

1 cup of Greek yogurt

½ tsp of fresh ginger, grated

1 tbsp of lemon juice

1 tbsp of chia seeds

1 tsp of cocoa powder

Preparation:

Combine oranges, carrot, lemon juice, ginger and chia seeds in a food processor. Blend until nicely smooth. Now, add yogurt and re-blend for 1 minute. Transfer the mixture to a serving glasses and sprinkle with cocoa. Refrigerate for 30 minutes before serving.

Nutrition information per serving: Kcal: 121, Protein: 8.2g, Carbs: 20.1g, Fats: 1.6g

39.   Spicy Turkey with Eggplant Puree

Ingredients:

2 lbs of turkey breasts, skinless and boneless

5 oz of cream cheese

2 tbsp of olive oil

2 tbsp of lemon juice

2 tbsp of green chili pepper, finely chopped

2 garlic clove, minced

1 tsp of fresh rosemary, finely chopped

½ tsp of sea salt

¼ tsp of black pepper, ground

For eggplant puree:

1 large eggplant, peeled and chopped

2 tbsp of butter

1 cup of skim milk

2 tbsp of lemon juice

¼ cup of cream cheese

2 tbsp of all-purpose flour

1 tsp of salt

Preparation:

Place eggplant in a large bowl. Add milk and lemon juice. Coat well and set aside to soak for 15 minutes. Sprinkle with some salt to taste.

Melt the butter in a large skillet over a medium-high temperature. Add flour and cheese. Cook for 1 minute, or until cheese melts. Pour eggplant mixture into the pan and cook until slightly tender. Remove from the heat and let it cool for a while. Transfer the mixture to a food processor and blend until nicely smooth. Set aside.

Combine oil, lemon juice, garlic and chili peppers in a large glass bowl. Place meat and coat well using a spoon. Refrigerate for 1 hour to allow flavors to penetrate into the meat.

Preheat the grill to a medium-high temperature. Grill for about 7-10 minutes on each side until golden brown. Top with cheese and grill until cheese begins to melt. Remove from the grill and serve with eggplant puree.

Nutrition information per serving: Kcal: 239, Protein: 18.6g, Carbs: 10.2g, Fats: 13.8g

40.   African Peanut Butter Stew

Ingredients:

½ cup of peanut butter

2 cups of sweet potatoes, peeled and cubed

1 cup of tomatoes, diced

2 small onions, chopped

1 small zucchini, peeled and chopped

2 small bell peppers, chopped

2 cups of tomato juice

2 tbsp of vegetable oil

2 garlic cloves, crushed

2 tbsp of coriander, ground

1 small chili pepper, minced

1 small eggplant, chopped

1 cup of water

½ tsp of salt

Preparation:

Place sweet potatoes in a pot of boiling water. Cook until fork-tender and remove from the heat. Drain and set aside.

Preheat the oil in a large nonstick skillet over a medium-high temperature. Add garlic, onions, coriander, and chili pepper. Cook for about 1-2 minutes, or until onions translucent. Now, add eggplant, tomatoes, and 1 cup of water. Cover with a lid and reduce the heat. Simmer for about 10-15 minutes. Add peppers and zucchini. Cook for another 20 minutes, stirring occasionally. Gradually stir in peanut butter and tomato sauce and add sweet potatoes. Adjust the thickness with adding more water. Cook for 20 minutes, until potatoes are tender.

Nutrition information per serving: Kcal: 174, Protein: 5.2g, Carbs: 20.1g, Fats: 9.5g

41. Ricotta Beets Salad

Ingredients:

1 cup of Ricotta cheese, crumbled

2 cups of beets, trimmed and chopped

3 cups of arugula, trimmed and chopped

½ cup of orange juice, freshly squeezed

2 tbsp of extra-virgin olive oil

½ tsp of Himalayan salt

¼ tsp of red pepper, ground

Preparation:

Place the beets in a pot of boiling water. Cook until fork-tender and remove from the heat. Drain and set aside.

Combine orange juice, oil, salt, and pepper in a large bowl. Mix well and add beets. Coat well with marinade and set aside for 30 minutes.

In a separate bowl, combine cheese and arugula. Top with soaked beets. Sprinkle with some extra salt and pepper to taste and serve.

Nutrition information per serving: Kcal: 207, Protein: 9.2g, Carbs: 16.0g, Fats: 12.2g

42.   Chives Omelet

Ingredients:

6 large eggs

1 cup of chives, chopped

½ cup of Feta cheese, crumbled

1 tbsp of butter

½ tsp of salt

¼ tsp of black pepper, ground

Preparation:

Beat the eggs in a medium-sized bowl. Sprinkle with salt and pepper and whisk until fluffy. Add chives and whisk again to combine. Set aside.

Melt butter in a large nonstick pan over a medium-high temperature. pour the egg mixture and spread evenly. Cook for 2 minutes and flip the omelet. Add cheese and cook for about 2-3 minutes more, or until set. Fold the omelet in half and remove from the heat. Serve.

Nutrition information per serving: Kcal: 372, Protein: 25.1g, Carbs: 3.9g, Fats: 28.8g

43.   Guacamole Salmon

Ingredients:

2 lbs of salmon filets, skinless and boneless

2 small avocados, pitted and chopped

1 large tomato, chopped

1 small onion, chopped

3 tbsp of fresh coriander, chopped

3 garlic cloves, minced

½ tsp of salt

¼ tsp of black pepper, ground

2 tbsp of olive oil

1 tbsp of rosemary, roughly chopped

2 tbsp of lemon juice

Preparation:

Place salmon filets in a large bowl. Add 1 tablespoon of oil, rosemary, and lemon juice. Coat well and set aside to allow flavors to penetrate into the meat.

Combine avocados, tomato, onion, coriander, garlic, salt, and pepper in a food processor. Blend until pureed. Transfer to a serving plate and set aside.

Preheat the remaining oil in a large nonstick skillet over a medium-high temperature. Add meat and cook for 5 minutes on each side. Remove from the heat and transfer to a serving plate with guacamole. Add extra salt and pepper, if needed. Serve immediately.

Nutrition information per serving: Kcal: 294, Protein: 23.4g, Carbs: 6.8g, Fats: 20.5g

44.　Quick Chicken Stew

Ingredients:

1 whole chicken, (about 3 lbs)

10 oz of fresh broccoli, chopped

7 oz cauliflower florets, chopped

1 large onion, finely chopped

1 large potato, peeled and chopped

3 medium-sized carrots, sliced

1 large tomato, peeled and chopped

A handful of yellow wax beans, whole

A handful of fresh parsley, finely chopped

2 tbsp of olive oil

2 tsp of salt

½ tsp of black pepper, ground

1 tbsp of Cayenne pepper, ground

Preparation:

Clean the chicken and generously sprinkle with some salt.

Set aside.

Grease the bottom of a pressure pot with olive oil. Add finely chopped onion and stir-fry for 3-4 minutes and then add sliced carrot. Continue to cook for 5 more minutes.

Now add the vegetables, salt, black pepper, Cayenne pepper, and top with chicken. Add one cup of water and close the lid.

Cook for 45 minutes.

Nutrition information per serving: Kcal: 290, Protein: 31.4g, Carbs: 39.6g, Fats: 6.8g

45.   Shallot Omelet

Ingredients:

6 large eggs, beaten

4 tbsp of sour cream

1 tbsp of butter

1 cup of shallots, chopped

½ tsp of ginger, ground

½ tsp of salt

¼ tsp of black pepper

Preparation:

Combine eggs, salt, and pepper in a mixing bowl. Beat well with a fork and set aside.

Melt the butter in a large nonstick frying pan over a medium-high temperature. Add shallots and sour cream. Stir in the eggs mixture and cook for 3 minutes. sprinkle with ginger and flip the omelet. Cook for another 3 minutes and fold the omelet. Remove from the heat and serve immediately.

Nutrition information per serving: Kcal: 377, Protein: 21.8g, Carbs: 16.1g, Fats: 25.8g

JUICES

1.   Apple Basil Juice

Ingredients:

1 medium-sized Granny Smith's apple, cored

1 cup of fresh basil, chopped

2 cups of broccoli, chopped

1 cup of fennel, chopped

1 oz of water

Preparation:

Wash the apple and cut lengthwise in half. Remove the core and chop into small pieces. Set aside.

Rinse the basil thoroughly under cold running water. Drain and torn into small pieces. Set aside.

Wash the broccoli and trim off the outer leaves. Chop into small pieces and fill the measuring cup. Reserve the rest for later. Set aside.

Trim off the fennel stalks and outer wilted layers. Wash and chop the fennel into bite-sized pieces. Fill the measuring cup and reserve the rest for later. Set aside.

Now, combine apple, basil, broccoli, and fennel in a juicer and process until juiced. Transfer to a serving glass and stir in the water.

Refrigerate for 5 minutes before serving.

Nutrition information per serving: Kcal: 140, Protein: 7.7g, Carbs: 41.8g, Fats: 1.3g

2.   Blueberry Lemon Juice

Ingredients:

1 cup of blueberries

1 whole lemon

2 medium red bell peppers, chopped

1 large wedge of honeydew melon

Preparation:

Wash the blueberries under cold running water. Drain and set aside.

Peel the lemon and cut lengthwise in half. Set aside.

Wash the bell peppers and cut in half. Remove the seeds and chop into small pieces. Set aside.

Cut the honeydew melon lengthwise in half. Scoop out the seeds using a spoon. Cut the large wedges and peel them. Cut into small chunks and place in a bowl. Wrap the rest of the melon in a plastic foil and refrigerate.

Now, process blueberries, lemon, bell peppers, and honeydew melon in a juicer.

Transfer to serving glasses and add some ice.

Serve immediately.

Nutritional information per serving: Kcal: 202, Protein: 5.5g, Carbs: 59.3g, Fats: 1.7g

3.   Apple Orange Juice

Ingredients:

1 medium-sized Granny Smith's apple, cored

1 medium-sized orange, peeled

1 cup of celery, chopped

1whole kiwi, peeled

1 tbsp of liquid honey

¼ tsp of ginger, ground

Preparation:

Wash the apple and cut lengthwise in half. Remove the core and cut into bite-sized pieces. Set aside.

Peel the orange and divide into wedges. Cut each wedge in half and set aside.

Wash the celery and chop into small pieces. Fill the measuring cup and reserve the rest for later. Set aside.

Peel the kiwi and cut lengthwise in half. Set aside.

Now, combine celery, kiwi, apple, and orange in a juicer and process until juiced. Transfer to a serving glass and stir in the honey and ginger.

Refrigerate for 5 minutes before serving.

Enjoy!

Nutrition information per serving: Kcal: 172, Protein: 3.5g, Carbs: 51.2g, Fats: 1.1g

4.   Apple Celery Juice

Ingredients:

1 small Granny Smith's apple, cored

1 large celery stalk, chopped

1 tsp of aloe juice

1 cup of cucumber, sliced

1 medium-sized banana, sliced

Preparation:

Wash the apple and cut in half. Remove the core and cut into bite-sized pieces. Set aside.

Wash the celery stalk and chop into bite-sized pieces. Set aside.

Wash the cucumber and cut into thin slices. Fill the measuring cup and reserve the rest for later. Set aside.

Peel the banana and cut into chunks. Set aside.

Now, combine apple, cucumber, banana, and celery in a juicer. Process until juiced.

Transfer to a serving glass and stir in the aloe juice.

Add some crushed ice and refrigerate for 5 minutes before serving.

Nutrition information per serving: Kcal: 174, Protein: 2.7g, Carbs: 50.3g, Fats: 0.8g

5.   Tomato Basil Juice

Ingredients:

1 large tomato, chopped

1 cup of fresh basil, torn

1 large cucumber, sliced

½ tsp of dried oregano, ground

1 oz of water

Preparation:

Wash the tomato and place it in a medium bowl. Cut into small pieces and reserve the juice while cutting. Set aside.

Wash the basil thoroughly and torn with hands. Set aside.

Wash the cucumber and cut into thick slices. Set aside.

Now, process tomato, basil, and cucumber in a juicer. Transfer to serving glasses and stir in the reserved tomato juice and water.

Sprinkle with dried oregano for some extra taste and serve immediately.

Nutritional information per serving: Kcal: 67, Protein: 4.3g, Carbs: 18.6g, Fats: 0.8g

6.   Sweet Apricot Pear Juice

Ingredients:

1 cup of apricots, pitted and halved

1 small pear, chopped

1 tbsp of liquid honey

1 small Delicious apple, cored

1 whole lemon, peeled and halved

1 cup of fresh mint, torn

Preparation:

Wash the apricots and cut each lengthwise in half. Remove the pits and fill the measuring cup. Reserve the rest in the refrigerator for some other juice.

Wash the pear and cut in half. Remove the core and cut into small pieces. Set aside.

Wash the apple and cut lengthwise in half. Remove the core and chop into bite-sized pieces. Set aside.

Peel the lemon and cut lengthwise in half. Set aside.

Rinse the mint thoroughly under cold running water. Drain and torn into small pieces. Set aside.

Now, combine apricots, pear, apple, lemon, and mint in a juicer and process until well juiced. Transfer to a serving glass and add some ice before serving.

Enjoy!

Nutrition information per serving: Kcal: 217, Protein: 4.9g, Carbs: 68.5g, Fats: 1.5g

7.   Apple Coconut Juice

Ingredients:

1 large Granny smith apple, peeled and cored

½ cup of pure coconut water, unsweetened

1 cup of pumpkin cubes

1 large banana, peeled

¼ tsp of nutmeg, ground

1 tbsp of coconut sugar

Preparation:

Wash the apple and remove the core. Cut into bite-sized pieces and set aside.

Peel the pumpkin and cut in half. Scoop out the seeds using a spoon. Cut one large wedge and peel it. Cut into small chunks and set aside. Reserve the rest for later.

Peel the banana and cut into chunks. Set aside.

Now, process pumpkin, banana, and apple in a juicer. Transfer to serving glasses and stir in the coconut water, coconut sugar, and nutmeg. Refrigerate for 30 minutes before serving.

Nutritional information per serving: Kcal: 338, Protein: 4.6g, Carbs: 97.8g, Fats: 1.4g

8.   Grapefruit Cauliflower Juice

Ingredients:

1 whole grapefruit, peeled

1 cup of cauliflower, chopped

1 large orange, peeled

1 cup of pineapple chunks

¼ cup of pure coconut water, unsweetened

Preparation:

Peel the grapefruit and orange and divide into wedges. Set aside.

Trim off the outer leaves of cauliflower. Wash it and cut into small pieces. Reserve the rest in the refrigerator.

Cut the top of a pineapple and peel it using a sharp knife. Cut into small chunks. Reserve the rest of the pineapple in a refrigerator.

Now, process pineapple, grapefruit, orange, and cauliflower in a juicer.

Transfer to serving glasses and stir in the pure coconut water.

Add few ice cubes and serve immediately.

Nutritional information per serving: Kcal: 247, Protein: 6.5g, Carbs: 74g, Fats: 1g

9. Guava Cucumber Juice

Ingredients:

1 large guava, peeled

1 large cucumber

1 ripe avocado, pitted and peeled

1 large lime, peeled

2 oz of coconut water

Preparation:

Peel the guava and cut into small chunks. Set aside.

Wash the cucumber and cut into thick slices. Set aside.

Peel the avocado and cut in half. Remove the pit and cut into chunks. Set aside.

Peel the lime and cut lengthwise in half. Set aside.

Now, process avocado, guava, cucumber, and lime in a juicer. Transfer to serving glasses and stir in the coconut water.

Add some ice cubes or refrigerate for 5 minutes.

Nutrition information per serving: Kcal: 352, Protein: 7.6g, Carbs: 41.6g, Fats: 30.3g

10.   Celery Cherry Juice

Ingredients:

1 cup of celery, chopped

1 cup of cherries, pitted

1 cup of watermelon, diced

1 small ginger knob, peeled

1 oz of water

¼ tsp of cinnamon, ground

Preparation:

Wash the celery and cut into small pieces. Fill the measuring cup and reserve the rest for later. Set aside.

Rinse the cherries under cold running water using a colander. Drain and cut each in half. Remove the pits and set aside.

Cut the watermelon in half. Cut one large wedge and wrap the rest in a plastic foil and refrigerate. Dice the wedge and remove the pits. Fill the measuring cup and set aside.

Peel the ginger knob and cut into small pieces. Set aside.

Now, combine watermelon, celery, cherries, and ginger knob in a juicer and process until juiced. Transfer to a serving glass and stir in the water and cinnamon. Add some ice and serve immediately.

Nutrition information per serving: Kcal: 143, Protein: 3.4g, Carbs: 40.2g, Fats: 0.7g

11.   Apple Strawberry Juice

Ingredients:

1 small apple, cored

2 large strawberries, chopped

2 large bananas, peeled and chunked

1 cup of fresh mint, chopped

2 oz of water

Preparation:

Wash the apple and cut in half. Remove the core and cut into bite-sized pieces. Set aside.

Wash the strawberries and remove the stem. Cut into bite-sized pieces and set aside.

Peel the bananas and cut into small chunks. Set aside.

Wash the mint and roughly chop it. Fill the measuring cup and set aside.

Now, combine apple, strawberries, bananas, and mint in a juicer and process until juiced. Transfer to a serving glass and stir in the water.

Add some ice and serve immediately.

Nutrition information per serving: Kcal: 294, Protein: 4.5g, Carbs: 86.1g, Fats: 1.4g

12.   Grapefruit Parsley Juice

Ingredients:

1 whole grapefruit, peeled

4 cups of parsley, chopped

1 cup of cantaloupe, diced

2 cups of mustard greens, torn

¼ cup of water

Preparation:

Peel the grapefruit and divide into wedges. Set aside.

Wash the mustard greens and parsley. Torn with hands and set aside.

Cut the cantaloupe in half. Scoop out the seeds and flesh. Cut two wedges and peel them. Chop into chunks and set aside. Reserve the rest of the cantaloupe in a refrigerator.

Now, process cantaloupe, mustard greens, grapefruit, and parsley in a juicer.

Transfer to serving glasses and stir in the water.

Add some ice and serve immediately.

Nutritional information per serving: Kcal: 206, Protein: 13.5g, Carbs: 59.3g, Fats: 3g

13. Cranberry Blueberry Juice

Ingredients:

1 cup of fresh cranberries

1 cup of fresh blueberries

3 medium Zestar apples, cored

1 cup of fresh kale, torn

1 tbsp of liquid honey

Preparation:

Combine cranberries and blueberries in a colander and wash under cold running water. Drain and set aside.

Wash the apples and remove the core. Cut into bite-sized pieces and set aside.

Wash the kale thoroughly and torn with hands. Set aside.

Now, process cranberries, blueberries, apple, and kale in a juicer.

Transfer to serving glasses and stir in the honey. Add some ice or refrigerate before serving.

Nutrition information per serving: Kcal: 368, Protein: 5.6g, Carbs: 106g, Fats: 2.2g

14. Radish-Swiss Chard Juice

Ingredients:

1 large radish, chopped

1 cup of chard, torn

1 cup of asparagus

1 cup of avocado, chopped

1 large honeydew melon wedge

¼ cup of pure coconut water, unsweetened

Preparation:

Wash the radish and trim off the green parts. Cut into small pieces and set aside.

Wash the chard thoroughly and torn with hands. Set aside.

Wash the asparagus and trim off the woody ends. Set aside.

Peel the avocado and cut in half. Remove the pit and cut into chunks. Set aside.

Cut the honeydew melon lengthwise in half. Scoop out the seeds using a spoon. Cut the large wedges and peel them. Cut into small chunks and place in a bowl. Wrap the rest of the melon in a plastic foil and refrigerate.

Now, process radish, chard, asparagus, avocado, and melon in a juicer.

Transfer to serving glasses and refrigerate 10 minutes before serving.

Nutritional information per serving: Kcal: 275, Protein: 8g, Carbs: 35.2g, Fats: 21,9g

15.   Mango Lemon Juice

Ingredients:

1 cup of mango, cubed

1 large lemon, peeled

1 cup of fresh cherries, pitted

1 cup of watermelon, cubed

1 tbsp of liquid honey

2 oz of water

Preparation:

Peel the mango and cut into small chunks. Set aside.

Peel the lemon and cut lengthwise in half. Set aside.

Wash the cherries under cold running water. Drain and cut in half. Remove the pits and set aside.

Cut the watermelon lengthwise. For one cup, you will need about 1 large wedge. Peel and cut into chunks. Remove the seeds and set aside. Reserve the rest of the melon for some other juices.

Now, process cherries, mango, lemon, and watermelon in a juicer.

Transfer to serving glasses and add few ice cubes before serving.

Nutrition information per serving: Kcal: 288, Protein: 4.6g, Carbs: 68.3g, Fats: 1.3g

16.   Carrot Cucumber Juice

Ingredients:

1 large carrot, peeled and sliced

1 cup of cucumber, sliced

1 large wedge of honeydew melon, peeled and cubed

1 cup of Swiss chard, torn

1 small ginger knob, peeled

¼ tsp of turmeric, ground

2 oz of water

Preparation:

Wash and peel the carrot. Cut into thin slices and set aside.

Wash the cucumber and cut into thin slices. Fill the measuring cup and reserve the rest for later. Set aside.

Cut melon lengthwise in half. Scoop out the seeds and then wash. Cut one large wedge and peel it. Cut into small cubes and set aside.

Rinse the Swiss chard thoroughly under cold running water. Drain and torn into small pieces. Set aside.

Peel the ginger knob and cut into small pieces. Set aside.

Now, combine melon, Swiss chard, carrot, and cucumber in a juicer and process until juiced. Transfer to a serving glass and stir in the turmeric and water.

Refrigerate for 10 minutes before serving.

Nutrition information per serving: Kcal: 92, Protein: 2.6g, Carbs: 25.7g, Fats: 0.5g

17.   Pumpkin Carrot Juice

Ingredients:

1 cup of pumpkin, cubed

2 large carrots, sliced

2 cups of Brussels sprouts, halved

1 small ginger knob, peeled and chopped

1 oz of water

Preparation:

Cut the pumpkin in half and scoop out the seeds. For one cup, you'll need about one large wedge. Cut and peel. Chop into bite-sized pieces and fill the measuring cup. Wrap the rest of the pumpkin in a plastic foil and reserve in the refrigerator.

Wash and peel the carrots. Cut into thin slices and set aside.

Wash the Brussels sprouts and trim off the outer wilted layers. Cut each sprout in half and set aside.

Peel the ginger knob and chop it into small pieces. Set aside.

Now, combine pumpkin, carrots, Brussel sprouts, and ginger in a juicer and process until juiced. Transfer to a serving glass and stir in the water.

Add some ice and serve immediately.

Nutrition information per serving: Kcal: 127, Protein: 8.5g, Carbs: 38.2g, Fats: 1.1g

18.   Carrot Apple Juice

Ingredients:

1 large carrot, sliced

1 small Granny Smith's apple, cored and chopped

1 cup of mango, chunked

1 oz of coconut water

Preparation:

Wash and peel the carrot. Cut into bite-sized pieces and set aside.

Wash the apple and cut in half. Remove the core and cut into bite-sized pieces. Set aside.

Peel the mango and cut into chunks. Fill the measuring cup and reserve the rest for later.

Now, combine carrot, apple, and mango in a juicer. Process until juiced. Transfer to a serving glass and stir in the coconut water. Add some crushed ice and serve immediately.

Enjoy!

Nutrition information per serving: Kcal: 179, Protein: 2.6g, Carbs: 51.2g, Fats:1.1g

19.   Banana Milk Juice

Ingredients:

1 large banana, peeled

2 tbsp of milk

2 cups of blueberries

1 cup of black grapes

1 cup of fresh mint, torn

¼ tsp of cinnamon, ground

Preparation:

Wash the banana and cut into thin slices. Set aside.

Place the blueberries in a colander. Rinse well under cold running water and drain. Set aside.

Wash the grapes and remove the stems. Fill the measuring cup and reserve the rest in the refrigerator. Set aside.

Wash the mint thoroughly under cold running water. Drain and torn into small pieces. Set aside.

Now, combine blueberries, grapes, mint, and banana in a juicer and process until juiced. Transfer to a serving glass and stir in the milk and cinnamon.

Refrigerate for 5 minutes before serving.

Nutrition information per serving: Kcal: 326, Protein: 6.2g, Carbs: 93.4g, Fats: 2.1g

20.　　Kale Strawberry Juice

Ingredients:

1 cup of fresh kale, torn

1 cup of strawberries, fresh

½ tsp of ginger, ground

1 lemon, peeled

Preparation:

Wash the kale thoroughly and torn with hands. Set aside.

Wash the strawberries under cold running water. Drain and set aside.

Peel the lemon and cut lengthwise in half. Set aside.

Combine kale, strawberries, and lemon in a juicer and process until juiced.

Transfer to a serving glass and add some ice cubes before serving.

Enjoy!

Nutritional information per serving: Kcal: 120, Protein: 5.9g, Carbs: 38.6g, Fats: 1.8g

21.　Tomato Mustard Green Juice

Ingredients:

1 medium-sized Roma tomato, chopped

1 cup of mustard greens, torn

2 cups of Romaine lettuce, chopped

1 cup of parsley, torn

1 whole cucumber, sliced

¼ tsp of turmeric, ground

¼ tsp of salt

Preparation:

Wash the tomato and place in a bowl. Chop into bite-sized pieces and reserve the tomato juice while cutting. Set aside.

Combine mustard greens and parsley in a large colander. Rinse well and drain. Torn into small pieces and set aside.

Rinse the lettuce thoroughly under cold running water. Chop into small pieces and set aside.

Wash the cucumber and cut into thin slices. Set aside.

Now, combine lettuce, tomato, mustard greens, parsley, and cucumber in a juicer and process until juiced. Transfer to a serving glass and stir in the turmeric, salt, and reserved tomato juice.

Refrigerate for 10 minutes before serving.

Enjoy!

Nutrition information per serving: Kcal: 85, Protein: 7.6g, Carbs: 25.3g, Fats: 1.6g

22.   Beet Apple Juice

Ingredients:

1 cup of beets, sliced

1 small Granny Smith's apple, cored

1 cup of fresh kale, torn

1 cup of cantaloupe, cubed

¼ tsp of ginger, ground

Preparation:

Wash the beets and trim off the green ends. Cut into thin slices and fill the measuring cup. Reserve the rest for some other juice.

Wash the apple and cut lengthwise in half. Remove the core and cut into bite-sized pieces. Set aside.

Rinse the kale thoroughly under cold running water. Drain and torn into small pieces. Set aside.

Cut the cantaloupe in half. Scrape out the seeds and cut one large wedge. Peel and chop into small pieces. Fill the measuring cup and wrap the rest in a plastic foil. Refrigerate for later.

Now, combine beets, apple, kale, and cantaloupe in a juicer and process until juiced. Transfer to a serving glass and stir in the ginger.

Add some ice and serve immediately.

Nutrition information per serving: Kcal: 181, Protein: 7g, Carbs: 51.1g, Fats: 1.4g

23.   Orange Apple Juice

Ingredients:

1 large orange, peeled

1 small Granny Smith's apple, cored

1 cup of papaya, chopped

1 cup of fresh mint, torn

1 tbsp of fresh basil, torn

Preparation:

Peel the orange and divide into wedges. Cut each wedge in half and set aside.

Wash the apple and cut in half. Remove the core and cut into bite-sized pieces. Set aside.

Wash and peel the papaya. Cut lengthwise in half and scoop out the seeds. Cut into bite-sized pieces and fill the measuring cup. Reserve the rest in the refrigerator.

Rinse the mint and basil thoroughly under cold running water. Drain and torn into small pieces. Set aside.

Now, combine orange, apple, papaya, mint, and basil in a juicer and process until juiced. Transfer to a serving glass and add some ice.

Serve immediately and enjoy!

Nutrition information per serving: Kcal: 199, Protein: 4.1g, Carbs: 60.1g, Fats: 1.1g

24.   Pumpkin Cinnamon Juice

Ingredients:

10 ozof sweet pumpkin chunks

½ tsp of cinnamon, freshly ground

1 cup of avocado chunks

¼ cup of water

Preparation:

Peel the pumpkin and cut in half. Scoop out the seeds using a spoon. Cut one large wedge and peel it. Cut into small chunks and set aside. Reserve the rest for later.

Peel the avocado in half. Remove the pit and cut into small chunks. Set aside.

Now, combine avocado and pumpkin in a juicer and process until juiced.

Transfer to serving glasses and stir in the water and cinnamon.

Add some ice before serving and enjoy!

Nutritional information per serving: Kcal: 256, Protein: 5.3g, Carbs: 27.8g, Fats: 22.3g

25.   Leek Asparagus Juice

Ingredients:

1 whole leek, chopped

2 medium-sized asparagus spears

1 cup of avocado, cubed

1 medium-sized zucchini

3 tbsp of water

Preparation:

Wash the leek and cut into small pieces. Set aside.

Wash the asparagus and trim off the woody ends. Cut into small pieces and set aside.

Peel the avocado and cut lengthwise in half. Remove the core and cut into small cubes. Fill the measuring cup and reserve the rest in the refrigerator.

Peel the zucchini and cut into bite-sized pieces. Set aside.

Now, combine avocado, zucchini, leek, and asparagus in a juicer and process until juiced. Transfer to a serving glass and stir in the water. Refrigerate for 10 minutes before serving.

Nutrition information per serving: Kcal: 277, Protein: 22.9g, Carbs: 32.7g, Fats: 22.9g

26. Blackberry Cinnamon Juice

Ingredients:

1 cup of blackberries

¼ tsp of cinnamon, ground

1 cup of cantaloupe, chopped

1 large orange, peeled

1 cup of fresh mint, torn

Preparation:

Place the blackberries in a colander and rinse well. Drain and set aside.

Cut the cantaloupe in half. Scrape out the seeds and cut one large wedge. Peel and chop into small pieces. Fill the measuring cup and wrap the rest in a plastic foil. Refrigerate for later.

Peel the orange and divide into wedges. Cut each wedge in half and set aside.

Rinse the mint under cold running water and drain. Torn into small pieces and set aside.

Now, combine and blackberries, cantaloupe, orange, and mint in a juicer and process until juiced. Transfer to a serving glass and stir in the cinnamon.

Add some ice and refrigerate for 5 minutes before serving.

Nutrition information per serving: Kcal: 157, Protein: 5.9g, Carbs: 51.9g, Fats: 1.5g

27.   Apricot Cucumber Juice

Ingredients:

1 cup of apricots, pitted

1 large cucumber

1 large peach, pitted

1 large apple, cored

1-inch piece of ginger root

Preparation:

Wash the peach and apricots. Cut in half andremove the pit. Cut into bite-sized pieces and set aside.

Wash the cucumber and cut into thick slices. Set aside.

Wash the apple and remove the core. Cut into bite-sized pieces and set aside.

Peel the ginger and set aside.

Now, combine apricots, peach, cucumber, apple, and ginger in a juicer. Process until juiced. Transfer to serving glasses and add some ice.

Serve immediately.

Nutrition information per serving: Kcal: 257, Protein: 6.7g, Carbs: 73.3g, Fats: 1.8g

28.   Carrot Cabbage Juice

Ingredients:

1 cup of carrots, sliced

1 cup of purple cabbage, chopped

1 cup of cauliflower, chopped

1 cup of collard greens, chopped

Preparation:

Wash the cauliflower and trim off the outer leaves. Cut into bite-sized pieces and fill the measuring cup. Reserve the rest for later.

Wash and peel the carrots. Cut into thin slices and fill the measuring cup. Set aside.

Combine cabbage and collard greens in a colander. Wash thoroughly under cold running water and slightly drain. Chop into small pieces and set aside.

Now, combine carrots, cabbage, cauliflower, and collard greens in a juicer and process until juiced. Transfer to a serving glass and refrigerate for 5 minutes before serving.

Nutrition information per serving: Kcal: 138, Protein: 5.3g, Carbs: 40.3g, Fats: 0.8g

29.   Celery Cucumber Juice

Ingredients:

2 celery stalks

1 large cucumber

3 large tomatoes

2 large carrots, sliced

1 bunch of fresh spinach

1 large bell pepper

Preparation:

Wash the celery and cucumber and chop into small pieces. Set aside.

Wash the tomatoes and place them in a bowl. Cut into small pieces and reserve the tomato juice while cutting. Set aside.

Wash the carrots and slice into a bowl with tomatoes.

Wash the bell pepper and cut in half. Remove the seeds and chop into small pieces.

Wash the spinach thoroughly and roughly chop it. Set aside.

Now, process tomatoes, carrots, celery, cucumber, spinach, and bell pepper in a juicer. Transfer to serving glasses and add the juices from the bowl.

Garnish with some fresh mint, but this is optional.

Refrigerate for 5 minutes before serving.

Enjoy!

Nutritional information per serving: Kcal: 248, Protein: 3.71g, Carbs: 70.5g, Fats: 3.71g

30.   Apple Mint Juice

Ingredients:

1 small apple, peeled and seeds removed

1 tsp of fresh mint leaves, finely chopped

1 cup of pineapple chunks

¼ tsp of nutmeg, ground

Preparation:

Wash the apple and remove the core. Cut into bite-sized pieces and set aside.

Garnish with mint leaves and refrigerate before serving.

Cut the top of a pineapple and peel it using a sharp knife. Cut into small chunks. Reserve the rest of the pineapple in a refrigerator.

Process pineapple and apple in a juicer. Transfer to a serving glasses and stir in the nutmeg. Add more water to increase the juice amount.

Nutritional information per serving: Kcal: 141, Protein: 1.5g, Carbs: 41.2g, Fats: 0.4g

31.   Orange Lettuce Juice

Ingredients:

1 large orange, peeled

1 cup of Romaine lettuce, shredded

1 cup of watermelon, peeled and seeded

1 cup of pomegranate seeds

Preparation:

Peel the orange and divide into wedges. Set aside.

Wash the lettuce thoroughly. Roughly chop it using hands and add set aside.

Cut the watermelon lengthwise. For one cup, you will need about one large wedge. Peel and cut into chunks. Remove the seeds and set aside.

Cut the top of the pomegranate fruit using a sharp knife. Slice down to each of the white membranes inside of the fruit. Pop the seeds into a medium bowl.

Now, process watermelon, orange, lettuce and pomegranate seeds in a juicer. Transfer to serving glasses and refrigerate for 5 minutes.

Nutritional information per serving: Kcal: 142, Protein: 5.2g, Carbs: 44.8g, Fats: 1.5g

32. Parsnip Orange Juice

Ingredients:

1 cup of parsnip, sliced

1 small orange, peeled

1 large peach, peeled

3 cups of red leaf lettuce, torn

1 tsp of agave syrup

Preparation:

Wash the parsnips and cut into thick slices. Set aside.

Peel the orange and divide into wedges. Set aside.

Wash the peach and cut in half. Remove the pit and cut into bite-sized pieces. Set aside.

Wash the lettuce thoroughly and torn it using hands. Set aside.

Now, process parsnips, orange, peach, and lettuce in a juicer. Transfer to serving glasses and stir in the agave syrup.

Add some ice and serve immediately.

Nutritional information per serving: Kcal: 177, Protein: 5.2g, Carbs: 53.7g, Fats: 1.1g

33. Carrot Parsnip Juice

Ingredients:

3 large carrots, sliced

1 cup of parsnips, sliced

2 large green apples, peeled and cored

1 basil leaf, crushed

¼ cup of water

Preparation:

Wash the carrots and parsnips and cut into thick slices. Set aside.

Wash the apples and remove the core. Cut into bite-sized pieces and set aside.

Now, combine apples, carrots, and parsnips in a juicer and process until juiced.

Transfer to serving glasses and stir in the water. Garnish with basil leaves and refrigerate before serving.

Enjoy!

Nutritional information per serving: Kcal: 332, Protein: 5.4g, Carbs: 100g, Fats: 1.6g

34.   Mango Ginger Juice

Ingredients:

1 cup of mango, chunked

1 small ginger slice

1 cup of pomegranate seeds

1 medium-sized apple, cored

¼ tsp of cinnamon, ground

1 oz of water

Preparation:

Peel the mango and cut into chunks. Fill the measuring cup and reserve the rest in the refrigerator. Set aside.

Peel the ginger slice and chop into small pieces. Set aside.

Cut the top of the pomegranate fruit using a sharp paring knife. Slice down to each of the white membranes inside of the fruit. Pop the seeds into a measuring cup and set aside.

Wash the apple and cut lengthwise in half. Remove the core and cut into small pieces. Set aside.

Now, combine pomegranate seeds, apple, mango, and ginger in a juicer and process until juiced. Transfer to a serving glass and stir in the cinnamon and water.

Refrigerate for 5 minutes before serving.

Nutrition information per serving: Kcal: 227, Protein: 3.6g, Carbs: 64.1g, Fats: 1.9g

35.   Cucumber Spinach Juice

Ingredients:

1 large cucumber, sliced

1 cup of fresh spinach, torn

1 cup of pineapple chunks

1 cup of apricots

1 whole lemon

½ cup of raw broccoli, chopped

½ cup of pure coconut water

Preparation:

Wash the cucumber and chop into thick slices. Set aside.

Peel the lemon and cut lengthwise in half. Set aside.

Combine spinach and broccoli in a colander and wash under cold running water. Drain and roughly chop. Set aside.

Cut the top of a pineapple and peel it using a sharp knife. Cut into small chunks. Reserve the rest of the pineapple in a refrigerator.

Wash the apricots and cut in half. Remove the pit and chop into chunks. Set aside.

Now, process cucumber, lemon, spinach, pineapple, apricots, and broccoli in a juicer. Transfer to serving glasses and stir in the coconut water.

Add some ice and serve immediately.

Nutritional information per serving: Kcal: 218, Protein: 10g, Carbs: 64g, Fats: 1.9g

36.   Lime Swiss Chard Juice

Ingredients:

1 whole lime, peeled

1 cup of chard, torn

1 cup of mango chunks

1 cup of beet greens, torn

½ cup of coconut water, unsweetened

Preparation:

Peel the lime and cut lengthwise in half. Set aside.

Combine chard and beet greens in a colander and wash under cold running water. Drain and torn with hands. Set aside.

Peel the mango and cut into small chunks. Set aside.

Now, combine lime, chard, mango, and beet greens in a juicer. Transfer to serving glasses and stir in the coconut water.

Add some ice or refrigerate for 5 minutes.

Enjoy!

Nutritional information per serving: Kcal: 108, Protein: 3.8g, Carbs: 33g, Fats: 0.8g

37.   Pepper Broccoli Juice

Ingredients:

1 small red bell pepper, seeded

1 small green bell pepper, seeded

1 small yellow bell pepper, seeded

1 cup of broccoli

1 cup of fresh kale

1 oz of water

Preparation:

Wash the bell peppers and cut in half. Remove the seeds and chop into small pieces. Set aside.

Wash the broccoli and kale in a colander under cold running water. Chop into small pieces and set aside.

Now, process peppers, broccoli, and kale in a juicer. Transfer to serving glasses and add a pinch of Cayenne pepper if you like it spicier. However, this is optional.

Serve immediately.

Nutritional information per serving: Kcal: 114, Protein: 8.7g, Carbs: 31.5g, Fats: 1.7g

38.   Apple Artichoke Juice

Ingredients:

1 Granny Smith apple, peeled and cored

1 large artichoke, chopped

1 cup of mustard greens, chopped

1 cup of Brussels sprouts

½ tsp of cinnamon, freshly ground

½ cup of pure coconut water, unsweetened

1 tsp of agave nectar

Preparation:

Wash the apple and remove the core. Cut into bite-sized pieces and set aside.

Using a sharp knife, trim off the outer leave of the artichoke. Cut into small pieces and set aside.

Wash the mustard greens and chop with hands. Set aside.

Wash the Brussels sprouts and trim off the outer layers. Set aside.

Now, process mustard greens, apple, artichoke, and

Brussels sprouts in a juicer.

Transfer to serving glasses and stir in the cinnamon, coconut water, and agave nectar.

Add some ice and serve immediately.

Nutritional information per serving: Kcal: 195, Protein: 13.7g, Carbs: 63.4g, Fats: 1.3g

39.   Cucumber Turmeric Juice

Ingredients:

1 cup of cucumber, sliced

¼ tsp of turmeric, ground

1 cup of crookneck squash, cubed

1 cup of pumpkin, chopped

¼ tsp of salt

2 tbsp of water

Preparation:

Wash the cucumber and cut into thin slices. Fill the measuring cup and reserve the rest in the refrigerator.

Cut the squash lengthwise in half. Using a teaspoon, scoop out the seeds and clean it inside. Peel and cut into small cubes. Fill the measuring cup and wrap the rest in a plastic foil and refrigerate.

Peel the pumpkin and cut lengthwise in half. Scoop out the seeds and cut into small cubes. Fill the measuring cup and reserve the rest in the refrigerator.

Now, combine cucumber, squash, and pumpkin in a juicer

and process until juiced. Transfer to a serving glass and stir in the turmeric, salt, and water.

Refrigerate for 5 minutes before serving.

Nutrition information per serving: Kcal: 73, Protein: 4.1g, Carbs: 19.3g, Fats: 0.9g

40.   Almond Honey Juice

Ingredients:

1 large banana, peeled

3 large red oranges, peeled

½ cup of almond milk, sugar-free

1 tbsp of honey, raw

1 tbsp of fresh mint leaves, finely chopped

Preparation:

Peel the banana and cut into small chunks. Set aside.

Peel the oranges and divide into wedges. Set aside.

Process banana and oranges in a juicer. Transfer to serving glasses and stir in the almond milk and honey.

Garnish with mint and refrigerate for 5 minutes before serving.

Enjoy!

Nutritional information per serving: Kcal: 411, Protein: 11g, Carbs: 95g, Fats: 3.1g

41.   Guava Swiss Chard Juice

Ingredients:

1 cup of pineapple chunks

1 whole guava, chopped

2 cups of chard, chopped

2 whole lemons, peeled

½ cup of coconut water, unsweetened

Preparation:

Wash the guava and cut into chunks. If you are using large fruit, reserve the rest for some other recipe in a refrigerator.

Wash the chard thoroughly under cold running water and set aside.

Cut the top of a pineapple and peel it using a sharp knife. Cut into small chunks. Reserve the rest of the pineapple in a refrigerator.

Peel the lemons and cut lengthwise in half. Set aside.

Now, process guava, chard, pineapple, and lemons in a juicer. Transfer to serving glasses and stir in the coconut water.

Add some ice and serve immediately.

Nutritional information per serving: Kcal: 130, Protein: 4.8g, Carbs: 43g, Fats: 1.2g

42.   Mustard Green Apple Juice

Ingredients:

1 cup of mustard greens, chopped

1 small Granny Smith's apple, cored

1 large wedge of honeydew melon, chopped

1 cup of fresh mint, chopped

1 oz of water

Preparation:

Combine mint and mustard greens in a colander and wash thoroughly. Slightly drain and chop into small pieces. Set aside.

Cut the melon in half. Cut one large wedge and peel the peel it. Cut into small pieces and set aside. Wrap the rest of the melon in a plastic foil and refrigerate for later.

Wash the apple and cut lengthwise in half. Remove the core and cut into bite-sized pieces. Set aside.

Now, combine mint, mustard greens, melon, and apple in a juicer and process until juiced.

Transfer to a serving glass and stir in the water. Refrigerate for 5 minutes before serving.

Nutrition information per serving: Kcal: 139, Protein: 4.1g, Carbs: 40.5g, Fats: 0.9g

43.   Carrot Cabbage Juice

Ingredients:

1 cup of carrots, chopped

2 cups of green cabbage, shredded

2 kiwis, peeled

1 whole grapefruit, peeled

1 tbsp of honey, raw

Preparation:

Wash the carrots and cut into small pieces. Set aside.

Wash the cabbage thoroughly and roughly chop it using hands. Set aside.

Peel the kiwis and cut in half. Set aside.

Wash the grapefruit and cut into chunks. Set aside.

Now, process carrots, cabbage, kiwis, and grapefruit in a juicer. Transfer to serving glasses and stir in the honey.

Add some ice cubes and serve immediately.

Nutritional information per serving: Kcal: 219, Protein: 6.9g, Carbs: 69g, Fats: 1.5g

44.   Carrot Cucumber Juice

Ingredients:

1 large carrot, sliced

1 cup of cucumber, sliced

1 cup of sweet potatoes, chunked

1 ginger knob, sliced

2 oz of water

Preparation:

Wash and peel the carrot. Cut into thin slices and set aside.

Wash the cucumber and cut into thin slices. Fill the measuring cup and reserve the rest for later.

Peel the potato and cut into small chunks. Fill the measuring cup and reserve the rest for later. Set aside.

Peel the ginger knob and cut into thin slices. Set aside.

Now, combine potato, ginger, carrot, and cucumber in a juicer and process until juiced transfer to a serving glass and stir in the water.

Nutrition information per serving: Kcal: 132, Protein: 3.2g, Carbs: 36.6g, Fats: 0.4g

45.   Cucumber Cantaloupe Juice

Ingredients:

1 large cucumber

1 cup of cantaloupe, cubed

1large honeydew melon wedge

1 cup of watermelon, seeded

1 tbsp of liquid honey

1 tbsp coconut water

Preparation:

Wash the cucumber and cut into thick slices. Set aside.

Cut the cantaloupe in half. Scoop out the seeds and flesh. Cut two wedges and peel them. Chop into chunks and set aside. Reserve the rest of the cantaloupe in a refrigerator.

Cut the honeydew melon lengthwise in half. Scoop out the seeds using a spoon. Cut one large wedge and peel. Cut into small chunks and place in a bowl. Wrap the rest of the melon in a plastic foil and refrigerate.

Cut the watermelon lengthwise. For one cup, you will need about 1 large wedge. Peel and cut into chunks. Remove the seeds and set aside. Reserve the rest of for some other juices.

Now, process cucumber, cantaloupe, honeydew melon, and watermelon in a juicer.

Transfer to serving glasses and stir in the honey and coconut water. Add some ice before serving.

Enjoy!

Nutritional information per serving: Kcal: 201, Protein: 3.4g, Carbs: 57.6g, Fats: 0.8g

46.   Pineapple Mint Juice

Ingredients:

1 cup of pineapple, chunked

1 cup of fresh mint, torn

1 cup of cucumber, sliced

1 whole guava, chopped

1 oz of water

Preparation:

Cut the top of the pineapple and peel it using a sharp paring knife. Peel it and cut into small pieces. Set aside.

Wash the mint and slightly drain. Torn with hands and set aside.

Wash the cucumber and cut into thin slices. Fill the measuring cup and reserve the rest in the refrigerator.

Wash and peel the guava fruit. Chop into bite-sized pieces and set aside.

Now, combine pineapple, mint, cucumber, and guava in a juicer and process until juiced. Transfer to a serving glass and stir in the water.

Refrigerate for 5 minutes before serving.

Nutrition information per serving: Kcal: 115, Protein: 3.6g, Carbs: 35.2g, Fats: 1.1g

47.   Broccoli Swiss Chard Juice

Ingredients:

1 cup of fresh broccoli, chopped

1 cup of Swiss chard, chopped

1 medium-sized artichoke, chopped

1 cup of cucumber, sliced

1 oz of water

Preparation:

Wash the broccoli and cut into small pieces. Fill the measuring cup and reserve the rest for later. Set aside.

Rinse the Swiss chard under cold running water. Slightly drain and chop into small pieces. Fill the measuring cup and reserve the rest in the refrigerator.

Trim off the outer leaves of the artichoke using a sharp paring knife. Wash it and cut into bite-sized pieces. Set aside.

Wash the cucumber and cut into thin slices. Fill the measuring cup and reserve the rest in the refrigerator. Set aside.

Now, combine artichoke, broccoli, Swiss chard, and cucumber in a juicer and process until juiced. Transfer to a serving glass and stir in the water.

Refrigerate for 5 minutes before serving.

Nutrition information per serving: Kcal: 65, Protein: 7.7g, Carbs: 22.7g, Fats: 0.6g

48.   Beet Cauliflower Juice

Ingredients:

1 cup of beets, trimmed

1 cup of beet greens, chopped

1 small cauliflower head

1 cup of parsnips, chopped

2 tbsp of fresh parsley

Preparation:

Wash the beets and trim off the green parts. Cut into small pieces. Chop the greens and set aside.

Trim off the outer leaves of a cauliflower. Wash it and chop into small pieces. Set aside.

Wash the parsnips and cut into thick slices. Set aside.

Now, process parsnips, beets, beet greens, and cauliflower in a juicer.

Transfer to serving glasses and refrigerate for 5 minutes. Garnish with fresh parsley before serving.

Nutritional information per serving: Kcal: 166, Protein: 9.9g, Carbs: 52.3g, Fats: 1.5g

49.   Radish Mint Juice

Ingredients:

1 medium-sized radish, chopped

1 tbsp of fresh mint, chopped

1 cup of cantaloupe, diced

1 cup of beet greens

1 cup of cauliflower, chopped

Preparation:

Wash the radish and trim off the green parts. Cut into small chunks and set aside.

Trim off the outer leaves of cauliflower. Wash it and cut into small pieces. Reserve the rest in the refrigerator.

Soak the mint leaves in water. Let it stand for about 2-3 minutes.

Cut the cantaloupe in half. Scoop out the seeds and flesh. Cut two wedges and peel them. Chop into chunks and set aside. Reserve the rest of the cantaloupe in a refrigerator.

Wash the beet greens and torn with hands. Set aside.

Now, process cantaloupe, beet greens, radish, cauliflower and mint in a juicer.

Transfer to serving glasses and add some ice before serving.

Nutritional information per serving: Kcal: 123, Protein: 8.1g, Carbs: 37.7g, Fats: 1.1g

ADDITIONAL TITLES FROM THIS AUTHOR

70 Effective Meal Recipes to Prevent and Solve Being Overweight: Burn Fat Fast by Using Proper Dieting and Smart Nutrition

By

Joe Correa CSN

48 Acne Solving Meal Recipes: The Fast and Natural Path to Fixing Your Acne Problems in Less Than 10 Days!

By

Joe Correa CSN

41 Alzheimer's Preventing Meal Recipes: Reduce or Eliminate Your Alzheimer's Condition in 30 Days or Less!

By

Joe Correa CSN

70 Effective Breast Cancer Meal Recipes: Prevent and Fight Breast Cancer with Smart Nutrition and Powerful Foods

By

Joe Correa CSN

www.ingramcontent.com/pod-product-compliance
Lightning Source LLC
Chambersburg PA
CBHW030249030426
42336CB00009B/312